Whole Foods Plant Based Diet

A Beginner's Guide to a Whole Foods Plant Based Diet

Gabby Roles

The Whole Foods Plant Based Diet: A Beginner's Guide to a Whole Foods Plant Based Diet

Gabby Roles

© 2013 by Gabby Roles

All Rights Reserved. No part of this publication may be reproduced in any form or by any means, including scanning, photocopying, or otherwise without prior written permission of the copyright holder.

This publication is designed to provide accurate and authoritative information in regard to the subject matter covered. It is sold understanding that the author/publisher is not engaged in rendering legal, accounting, medical or other professional services.

The information and opinions presented in this book are intended for educational purposes only and are not to be used for diagnosis and treatment, or a substitute for professional medical advice. In the case of a need for such expertise consult with the appropriate professional.

ISBN-13:

978-0615865614 (CKB Publishing)

ISBN-10:

0615865615

Contents

Introduction 5

The Definition of Whole Foods 8

The Reasons to Choose Whole Foods 14

Whole Foods are Better than Supplements 25

Avoid Nutrient Shortages 31

Why Active People Need Whole Foods 38

You Can Get Protein in a Plant Based Diet 42

How to Ease into a Plant Based Diet Slowly 46

Introduction

Whole foods plant based diets, contrary to popular belief, don't mean that you can only eat fruits and vegetables. This diet, which differs from a strictly vegetarian diet, is good for your body, skin and even the environment and simply means that a majority of the food you consume comes directly from whole, unprocessed food. There is still room for minimal amounts of lean meat and fish, but the main focus is on eating plant based foods.

Whole foods are those that are as close to the original source as possible. They are not processed and contain little to no additives including sugar, salt and artificial ingredients. These foods are unrefined and can be eaten in their natural state.

They require little to no modifications, which is why you are able to gain the benefit of close to 100 percent of the vital nutrients that the food has to offer. Whole foods reduce the likelihood of losing the vital nutrients in each type of food that occurs when they are processed or even in some methods of cooking.

If preventing the risk of diabetes, hypertension and heart disease are not enough for you to consider a whole foods diet, consider the fact that it could help you lose weight, keep your gastrointestinal system in check and even give you beautiful skin. All of these benefits are possible when the right diet is followed. There are no steadfast rules that you must follow and no risk of failing the diet. When you put your best foot forward and choose the right foods to eat on a regular basis, your health will benefit.

This book is meant to help you get a better understanding of what a whole foods diet can look like and to help you understand how you might be able to benefit from a few simple changes in your life. If a majority of your food consumption stems from convenience foods that come in a box and have a long shelf life, you might want to consider switching over to a more wholesome diet.

Convenience or processed food only serves to fill your body with higher than acceptable levels of sugar, salt and various useless additives that can actually harm your body.

The goal in this book is to guide you to start eating healthier, one step at a time. This is not a crash diet. It is a change in your lifestyle, a guide to help you make better food choices on a daily basis. It is not a diet that will fail if you "cheat" and give into a sweet tooth once in a while or quietly sneak that salty snack that you just can't live without.

This is a way of life, a way to help you live a happier, fuller and hopefully longer life. What you put into your health is what you take out of it, but the end result is a life with fewer medications, a lower body weight and a happier demeanor – it's a journey well worth taking.

The Definition of Whole Foods

Understanding Whole Foods

The first step to following a whole foods plant based diet is understanding what it means. To put it plain and simple, it means filling a majority of your diet with foods that are not processed or refined and come directly from plants. They are foods that are as close as possible to their original source and are completely unmodified. It is not a diet restricted solely to fruits and vegetables; there are many delicious alternatives to help you have a satisfying choice of foods to eat.

Get Your Phytochemicals

The only place to get phytochemicals is in whole foods, such as fruits, vegetables, beans and whole grains. These essential nutrients have a direct impact on your health.

The latest research determines that a few of the key phytochemicals might help to prevent certain cancers, lower cholesterol, keep the gastrointestinal tract healthy and protect various cells throughout the body. There are thousands of different forms available, but the most commonly known nutrients are terms that might be a little more familiar to you: flavonoids, antioxidants and carotenoids.

How do you fill your diet with these amazing nutrients? Start by creating a rainbow of colors on your plates. The more colorful fruits and vegetables that you consume, the higher the chances of consuming the nutrients your body needs.

There are many beautiful colored fruits and vegetables to choose from including red tomatoes, blue blueberries, orange carrots, pink watermelon, pink grapefruit, green spinach, green kale, red strawberries and red raspberries. The more colors on your plate, the more benefits you are providing your body.

In addition to fruits and vegetables, phytonutrients can be found in whole grain bread, whole grain cereal, walnuts, sunflower seeds, peas, lentils, green tea and black tea. If you do consume breads and cereals, it is important to ensure that they are truly made from whole grains, not processed grains which could be stripped of the nutrients you assume you are obtaining by eating it.

Is Organic A Requirement?

Eating whole foods does not mean that they must be locally grown or even organic; that is a completely different topic. This does not mean that your whole foods cannot be organic; it is just not a prerequisite to qualify as whole or natural. Obviously, organic or locally grown food could provide you with the added benefit of eliminating harmful toxins and chemicals, which can further the health benefit of eating whole foods.

Maximize Nutrients In Vegetables

The reason that we eat food, besides that it tastes good, is to obtain the vital nutrients necessary for good health. When you consume food that has been modified, processed or refined, the important nutrients are removed. This is even true for those foods that you consider healthy. For example, you might think you are doing your body good by eating spinach or broccoli. But if you do not eat it raw or prepare it properly, you are likely losing some of its nutrients, especially those that are water soluble. Vitamin B and C are two of the water soluble vitamins found in both vegetables that are lost when these vegetables are cooked in water, whether boiled or steamed. Choosing to eat these vegetables raw is the best way to consume all vital nutrients. If you prefer them cooked, choose methods such as sautéing, stir frying or blanching as each of these methods are considered "quick cooking" methods and avoid the risk of losing many nutrients.

Choosing Whole Grains

In addition to eating fruits and vegetables, a whole foods diet also includes eating a variety of whole grains. Care should be taken when you choose your grains, however. Not all whole grains are as "whole" as they sound. When you choose the right grains, you can reap the benefits of complex carbohydrates as well as vital vitamins and nutrients, adding taste, texture and proper nutrition to your diet.

Grains are found in the seeds of various grasses. They can be found in various forms including wheat, oats, rice, cornmeal and barley. When grains start out, they are considered whole and their most important ingredients bran and germ are intact.

It is during the processing of these grains that they are stripped of bran and germ as well as their vital nutrients. This is what results in refined and enriched grains, which make up the products that have a longer shelf life, such as white bread and white rice.

These foods, as you probably know, are less healthy for you. When you read product labels, look for the words refined or enriched grains and steer clear. In refined grains, the lost nutrients are never replaced.

In enriched grains, the products are fortified with the stripped nutrients, but it does not provide the same benefits as eating whole foods with the natural nutrients right from the start.

Creating the Perfect Meals

Creating the perfect meals with the right plant based whole foods does not have to be difficult. In fact, it is best to get creative in order to maximize the nutrients that you consume.

Start with the basics including whole grain breads, whole grain pasta, steel cut oats, colorful fruits and raw vegetables.

Then you can get creative:

- Add fruits and spices to your oatmeal
- Add flax seed to your whole grain cereal
- Make salad the main course for lunch or dinner and get creative
- Add your favorite vegetables to whole grain pasta or rice
- Make smoothies with as many fruits and vegetables as possible
- Add plant based, natural nut butters to whole grain bread
- Eat fruit for dessert
- Add beans to lunch and dinner entrées
- Include at least one fruit and vegetable at every meal

The Reasons to Choose Whole Foods

Everyone Has a Different Reason

There are a variety of reasons that people turn to a diet made of whole foods.

The most common reasons include the ability to help fight chronic illnesses, maintain a healthy weight and to fight the signs of aging. As an added bonus, some people have realized benefits that include:

- A feeling of wellness due to a reduction in the amount of chemicals consumed
- Better gastrointestinal health
- Reduced occurrences of depression

Fight Chronic Illnesses

Chronic illness has many different faces including cancer, heart disease, diabetes and hypertension. The one common factor that each of these illnesses has is a poor diet.

While this is not the singlehanded reason for every illness, it can contribute greatly to the risks. For most people, it is well worth the effort it takes to try a whole foods diet to try to prevent or even fight the presence of chronic illness.

The Facts Say It All

When you consider that more than three quarters of the nation's healthcare costs are to pay for treatment of chronic disease, the numbers speak for themselves.

Chronic disease is the leading cause of disability and death in our nation. What makes these numbers even worse is the fact that many of the diseases could have been prevented, rather than treated.

With more than 70 percent of American deaths being caused by chronic illness, it is time for Americans to learn the benefits of diets made of whole foods to prevent disease.

Heart Disease

Heart disease is the leading cause of death in the United States. Luckily, there are steps you can take to prevent your risks. While you cannot do anything about your genes and the diseases that you are predisposed to, changing your lifestyle can help to reduce the risks.

Your diet, what you do and do not eat, is the main factor in prevention. When you choose plant based whole foods, you are making a conscious effort to lower your cholesterol and reduce your blood pressure, which can help to reduce the risk of heart attack or stroke.

A majority of American's diets are laden with excessive amounts of fat, which can cause high cholesterol. When cholesterol builds up in the arteries, it can cause blocked arteries that result in heart disease including stroke and heart attack. Of utmost concern are trans fats, which are found in baked goods as well as fried and processed foods.

Trans fat not only increases your bad cholesterol, but also decreases the good cholesterol, putting your heart at even greater risk for disease. This is reason enough to make the choice to avoid butter, margarine and shortening in your diet. When you eliminate these fats from your diet, you might even realize how much you enjoy plant based whole foods.

Experiment at each meal with a variety of vegetables, eating them raw or lightly sautéed and savor the experience. When you avoid drenching your food in butter, sour cream and fattening dressing, you experience what food is supposed to taste like, not a processed mess.

Think about the amount of times you have loaded up your baked potato with butter and sour cream or weighed your salad down with fattening, additive filled dressings. You have masked what the food is actually supposed to taste like. Try to enjoy these natural foods by making a few simple changes to your meals in order to make your diet instantly healthy. A few of the best heart healthy foods include:

- Legumes - especially black beans or kidney beans
- Almonds
- Blueberries
- Broccoli

This is not an exhaustive list of course. You should incorporate as many fruits and vegetables as possible in each meal in order to reap the benefits of all of the heart healthy foods.

As a general rule of thumb, fill your plate two thirds full of fruits and vegetables in order to give your heart its best chance at preventing disease.

Cancer

More than 1.5 million Americans are diagnosed with cancer every year. Those are staggering numbers that should have every American scrambling to find out how they can prevent their chances of suffering from this often fatal disease. One of the largest factors is the lifestyle that most Americans lead.

Choosing whole foods that are plant based can help to dramatically decrease your risks, while choosing other foods that are not as healthy can actually cause cancer.

Making the switch to healthier foods can help to minimize your risks as well as give you an overall feeling of good health.

Lifestyle changes are among the most important decisions you can make to help fight your risk of cancer.

Everyone should try to eliminate any bad choices including:

- Smoking
- Drinking excessive amounts of alcohol
- Avoiding exercise
- Eating unhealthy

When you eliminate these behaviors from your lifestyle, you can then focus on the good behaviors and choices, which include eating foods that fight cancer, not fuel it. Choosing foods that are not processed and are as close to their natural source as possible is the best way to help your body.

Making small changes to your diet can have a huge impact on your overall health. Consider changes such as:

- Choosing potatoes over potato chips
- Eating apples rather than applesauce
- Adding nuts and cinnamon to your steel cut oatmeal rather than eating instant oatmeal
- Avoid creamy sauces, choosing to add fresh veggies or salsa to your dishes

Once you eliminate the "bad" foods from your diet, you can start to focus on those foods that contain the good properties that help to fight cancer including:

- **Antioxidants** - These essential vitamins help to protect your cells from damage from free radicals which is thought to be a cause of cancer. Choose from a variety of foods including berries, grapes, beans and carrots.

- **Phytochemicals** – There are literally thousands of these nutrients found in plant based foods that mimic the effects of antioxidants, helping to fight cancer. Consider consuming carrots, chick peas, broccoli and onions to obtain these benefits.

- **Polyphenols** – These are nutrients that are known to have anti-inflammatory properties which can help to protect cells against the risk of cancer and are found in blueberries, raspberries and onions, as well as others.

Maintain a Healthy Weight

Consider the difference between eating heavily processed, additive filled food and food directly from its source. Which one do you think will have fewer calories? It will always be the natural food that is eaten as it should, no butter, oil or fattening condiments.

All that processed food can do for you is cause you to gain weight, maintain an unhealthy weight and add to your risk of suffering from health issues, such as Type 2 diabetes and hypertension.

Switching to a plant based whole foods diet can quickly eliminate these risks as well as allow you to be the weight you were meant to be.

Eating more while dieting sounds pretty contradictory, doesn't it? But it's possible! If you enjoy food, you do not have to despair if you are considering a whole foods plant based diet. If you are looking at this process as a way to change your life, giving you a new way of eating from now on, not as a fad, you will enjoy the process and be able to eat more.

There are significantly fewer calories in plant based foods that are eaten as they are meant to be, than foods that are processed or cooked with fattening additives. This means that you can eat more food and still consume fewer calories!

As an added benefit, when you give your body the nutrients it needs by eating the right fruits and vegetables, your body will stop craving unnecessary calories. This means that it could be easier to stop overeating, which could result in a few lost pounds.

When you begin a whole foods plant based diet, you become more conscious about the food that you consume. Reading labels will quickly become a habit. You might be very surprised at the ingredients included in the foods that you once ate.

The levels of sodium, sugar and additives that have names you cannot even pronounce could be preventing you from maintaining a healthy weight. Becoming conscious about every bite you put in your mouth can help you become the healthy weight you desire and stay that way!

Keep Your Youthful Skin

As you age, it might seem inevitable that you start to show the signs on your face, neck and hands. The good news is that it is preventable! Believe it or not, the food that you consume has a direct impact on how your skin looks.

Eating animal products, fat and other additives only serve to clog pores, making your skin suffer. Just like in the world of medicine, there are creams and ways to hide the flaws on your skin, but is that how you want to live your life? What if you could have beautiful, glowing skin naturally?

Whole foods that are plant based are naturally devoid of any saturated fats. These fats that you find in meat, dairy and processed foods are what clog your pores, cause your skin to become inflamed and even cause acne.

When you eliminate these foods from your diet, you instantly give yourself a natural facial, without any procedures in a dermatologist's chair or the need for chemically filled medications. The right fruits and vegetables can provide the antioxidants and phytonutrients that are essential to smooth, glowing skin, no procedures necessary.

As an added benefit, plant based whole foods provide your body with necessary fiber. This enables your digestive system to work properly, which helps your body eliminate toxins that are obtained through the food you eat as well as the environment around you.

When you burden your body with too many toxins, your organs that are responsible for eliminating the toxins stop working effectively. This puts the job of toxin elimination on your skin, which as you guessed, leaves you with flaws that could have been prevented.

Whole Foods Are Better Than Supplements

Get the Real Nutrients

Many people make the mistake of assuming that they can take a supplement to make up for the nutrients they lack. While there are thousands of supplements available, they do not take the place of the nutrients straight from the source.

If you are consuming an unhealthy, calorie ridden diet filled with saturated fat, even the best supplements are not going to provide any benefit.

You could still be subjected to the risks of high blood pressure, heart disease, diabetes and cancer, even if you take supplements.

The Downfall of Supplements

The largest downfall of supplements is that they only provide one nutrient that you are lacking.

They do not provide the overall nutrition that whole foods can provide. Most fruits and vegetables provide a constant source of a variety of nutrients, not just one.

They are a complex combination of micronutrients that are necessary in order to work together to provide the nutrition that your body requires. The nutrients that you consume in food are provided in balanced proportions, unlike supplements.

In addition, they are offered in a way that is easier to digest, giving your body a better chance of reaping the benefits rather than wasting valuable nutrients.

Get Your Fiber

Fiber is a key component in any diet. It helps to regulate your digestive system, eliminate toxins from your body, maintain a healthy weight and even prevent disease.

Fiber is not available through the use of supplements, making it essential to vary your diet with many different colored fruits and vegetables to gain the required nutrients to maintain optimal health.

A Constant Interaction

Your diet as a whole is what determines your level of health and well-being. Taking one or two supplements might seem like a good idea, but they do not provide your body with the overall effect that food can provide.

For example, tomatoes are known for their abundance of Vitamin C, but did you know that they also provide Vitamin A, fiber, carbohydrates, phytochemicals and antioxidants?

These are benefits that cannot be obtained from supplements alone and would deprive your body of these crucial nutrients if chosen over whole foods.

Overdoing It

There is such a thing as too much of a good thing. High levels of certain nutrients can turn toxic in your body, which is another reason why getting your nutrients straight from the source is important.

Typically the nutrients found in foods are available in balanced amounts that make it difficult to overdo it on just one nutrient.

Supplements, on the other hand, can become toxic if too many are taken.

In addition, if you take supplements and are not aware of how they interact with other supplements you might be taking, you could reduce their effectiveness, depriving your body of the essential nutrients.

What You Can Do

Sometimes a complete diet makeover is essential to ensure that you are receiving the right nutrients. Take a close look at your overall diet. Is it filled with large amounts of convenience or drive-thru food? If so, it is time for a switch to plant based whole foods, not supplements in combination with your poor diet habits. Start with small changes such as:

- Fill your shopping cart with a variety of fruits and vegetables. You should see a rainbow of colors in your cart in order to obtain the most nutrients.

- Make general changes such as eating nutrient dense spinach in your salads rather than nutrient lacking iceberg lettuce or eating an apple rather than drinking sugar laden apple juice.

- Make conscious choices when you eat, don't just grab the first food that you find. This typically leads to eating highly processed food that offers zero nutritional value.

- Have plenty of variation in your diet. The more colors that you include, the more nutrients you give your body and the higher your chances of fighting disease.

Avoid Nutrient Shortages

In general, Americans consume too many calories. What's even more shocking about that? They still do not get enough nutrients!

More food does not equal more nutrients; in fact, it could mean even less nutrients if the food you are consuming is filled with preservatives and additives that actually harm the body.

Most of the food that a majority of us consume is filled with too much sugar, fat and sodium and none of the good things like Vitamin A, Vitamin C, calcium, potassium or fiber.

Filling the Gap

Just how do you fill the gap that you might be experiencing in your nutrition? Plant based whole foods are key. You must not stop there though; it is not enough to start consuming more of one or two fruits.

Your diet requires plenty of variation in order to maximize the number of nutrients that you obtain. It goes back to the same rule that was stated before, the more colorful your plate, the more nutrients you are obtaining.

A Change In Your Lifestyle

A mistake that many people make is assuming that a small cup of vegetables on the side of their otherwise, unhealthy or evening fattening dinner, will give them the nutrients that they need. A whole foods plant based diet puts fruits and vegetables at the forefront of the meal, not as an afterthought.

The main focus should be on the plant based foods that you can fill your plate with rather than meat and unhealthy carbohydrates. Consider foods with the highest level of nutrients including green leafy vegetables, bright orange sweet potatoes and a variety of legumes.

You can also include a healthy variety of whole grains, such as whole grain brown rice or whole grain pasta once in a while. It is important to ensure that each ingredient in these products is considered "whole" in order for it to count towards your plant based diet though.

Boost your Immune System

Are you one of those people that constantly has a cold or the flu in the winter?

Do family and friends look at you in amazement when you have to bow out of an obligation because of yet another illness?

Take a close look at your diet to see if you are lacking the most important nutrients, the ones that boost your immune system.

The more colorful the fruits and vegetables that you consume, the more antioxidants that you obtain, giving your body a fighting chance at avoiding numerous colds and the flu all year long.

The Crucial Nutrients

There are more than 30 essential nutrients that everybody needs in order to function as it was meant to operate. There are nutrients that are vital for growth, maintenance and protection and some that perform multiple duties. Consider Vitamin C and all of its duties:

- **Antioxidant** – Protects the body from free radical damage
- **Collagen Producer** – Helps wounds heal
- **Immune Booster** – Helps the immune system fight off disease

Foods to Consume

In order to fill your nutrient shortages, you should focus on the following foods to gain the nutrients that most commonly lack:

Vitamin A

- Green Leafy Vegetables
- Broccoli
- Carrots
- Squash
- Cantaloupe
- Mangos

Vitamin E

- Hazelnuts
- Almonds
- Sweet Potatoes
- Spinach
- Chickpeas
- Broccoli

Calcium

- Green Leafy Vegetables
- Broccoli
- Beans
- Whole Grains

Fiber

- Pumpkin Seeds
- Sunflower Seeds
- Pears
- Kiwi
- Blackberries
- Raspberries
- Apricots
- Beans

Potassium

- Swiss Chard
- Spinach
- Tomatoes
- Carrots
- Cauliflower
- Asparagus

Why Active People Need Whole Foods

Nutrition Enhances Exercise Efforts

If you are active, whether you run, weight lift or walk on a treadmill, you need optimal nutrition. Exercise is great, but without the right nutrients, your body does not reap all of the benefits.

What you eat before and after your exercise routines play a large role in what you get out of your efforts. Without optimal nutrition, or the right balance between macronutrients and micronutrients, you could be missing the benefits of your hard work.

Unrefined Carbohydrates

A mistake that many people make is assuming they need to load up on carbohydrates before working out. While carbohydrates are necessary, there is a difference between unrefined and refined carbs.

Rather than loading up on white pasta or white bread, you can choose to load up on fresh fruits, vegetables and whole grains. These carbs are also full of fiber which helps your body slowly digest them, keeping your blood sugar level in check.

Pre-Workout

What you eat before your workout is important, but not as important as what you eat after the fact. Between one and four hours before your intended activity, you should have a small amount of unrefined carbohydrates. This could simply mean a few pieces of fruit or a piece of whole grain bread with natural nut butter.

A small amount of carbohydrates and calories will be able to fuel your muscles through a basic workout. If your routine will be more intense, an increase in the amount you eat might be necessary.

A Quicker Recovery

As you work out on a regular basis, you are working your muscles hard, actually causing small tears throughout the muscle fibers. This is how muscle grows. But in order for your muscles to be able to react properly, they need rest time. This is evident in the level of soreness you feel in your muscles.

If you do not feed your body the right nutrients, you could be too sore to work out for quite a few days. This could make it difficult to build muscle if you can only work out once or twice a week. The right plant based whole foods can aid your muscles in their recovery, enabling you to work out more often.

Immediately following a workout, which means within the first 30-45 minutes afterwards, you should fuel your body with the right foods including the right carbohydrates and protein.

Your post-workout nutrition should look something like this:

- Immediately following exercise – Eat a piece of fruit

- Within the first hour – Eat a heavier meal including a combination between carbohydrates and protein. A few examples include: a sweet potato and green leafy salad or legumes and brown rice.

Hydration Is Important Too

Hydration is crucial before, during and after exercise. Water contains all of the nutrients you need while working out and will properly regulate your temperature, keep your joints loose and provide your body with the appropriate nutrients as you exercise.

Your muscles thrive on the hydration and need plenty of cool water before you even step foot in the gym. Consistently refuel your body with water every 20 minutes during the workout and continue for as long as possible after your workout.

Your body will tell you when you have or have not had enough hydration. A few of the signs of dehydration include:

- Cramps
- Dizziness or loss of balance
- Incredible fatigue

If you dislike the taste of plain water or get bored, you can add a few squeezes of fresh lemon to your water to give it a little taste as well as the added benefits of extra vitamins while you work out.

You Can Get Protein in a Plant Based Diet

The Importance of Protein

One worry that many people have when they consider going on a diet, whether it's plant based or otherwise, is the amount of protein they will consume.

While protein is one of three most important macronutrients that you need to take in on a daily basis, you can get it in many places that you might not even realize.

Most people meet their requirements simply by eating a varied diet without focusing on protein consumption.

More than Meat

Contrary to popular belief, meat is not the only place to get protein. In fact, most Americans consume 50 percent more protein than they need. This could put them at risk for serious illnesses as a result.

Unlike fat, your body cannot store protein. This means that when you consume too much of it, your body has to work overtime to get rid of it. This puts your liver and kidneys in overdrive and at risk for damage.

It also allows for an acidic buildup in your body which can cause health issues down the road and an over consumption of saturated fat which puts you at risk for heart disease and stroke.

What to Eat

Rather than focusing on the protein on your plate, try to fill your plate with variety. Remember the goal of making every meal look like a rainbow of colors? That's how you will get adequate, healthy protein.

All foods that come from plants contain the amino acids which are the building blocks of protein. Of course, there are certain vegetables that contain higher levels of the amino acids than others.

Try to focus your food choices on the following groups:

- Green leafy vegetables
- Broccoli
- Beans
- Steel cut oatmeal
- Whole grain rice
- Almonds
- Chickpeas
- Quinoa
- Peas
- Spinach

Determining Your Needs

Everyone has different needs for protein consumption. Children start out needing only around 13 grams of protein per day. As they grow, their protein needs increase.

By the time they are in their teen years, girls require around 46 grams and boys around 52 grams of protein.

Those numbers stay pretty steady as they head into adulthood, but some adults might require a few more grams, depending on their lifestyle.

If you are really active, you might have a greater need for protein, but not by a drastic amount. Focusing on a well-balanced diet will help you get the macronutrients that you need.

Consistent Variety

The best way to ensure that your body gets everything that it needs, not just protein, is to put your focus on a variety of plant based whole foods.

When your meals are varied and your food choices are whole, your body will obtain the right amount of amino acids.

As an added bonus, you will also get plenty of antioxidants, phytonutrients and fiber – all of which you would not get from animal protein.

How to Ease into a Plant Based Diet Slowly

You are What you Eat

If your diet is laden with foods that are heavily processed, contain an overabundance of sugar or salt or are very fattening, chances are you are not going to feel healthy.

The food you eat is what fuels your body. If you are not providing your body with the right nutrients, you might feel sluggish, unhappy and unhealthy.

This occurs because your body views the processed food and additives that you eat as toxins, which causes your body to react negatively.

If you want to feel healthy and happy, you should focus your food choices on whole foods. This is not as difficult as it sounds.

Starting Out

To determine what your body is doing, start by taking a close look at your current diet. Keep a food journal for a week, to allow yourself to see what it is that your body consumes on a daily basis.

Your journal should include:

- Food eaten at all meals, including all condiments such as butter, sour cream, dressing, syrup, etc...
- All snacks
- All beverages

Don't overlook anything that you consume; it all counts towards your calorie count as well as your nutritional values.

When you are conscious about what you are eating, you might realize that your diet is not as healthy as you once thought. Then you can determine how to start making changes.

The Foods To Eat

If you slowly start to replace your current diet with plant based foods that are direct from the source, you will begin to give your body what it craves. There are significantly fewer calories in a plate full of healthy vegetables, rather than a big, juicy steak that was cooked in butter with a loaded baked potato on the side.

Does this mean that you have to give up that steak dinner forever? No, it simply means that you need to learn to modify your food choices.

Once in a while it is okay to give into your cravings for a meat dinner; you just need to make different choices by cooking without butter or oils, avoid over cooking your vegetables to retain their nutrients and their taste and eliminating fattening condiments.

Start Slow

Take a look at your food journal and determine where to start. If you notice an overabundance of snacking going on throughout your days, you can start by cutting them out. This does not mean that you need to go hungry.

Swap those potato chips for cut up green peppers for the same crunch, yet less calories and more taste. If you need something sweet, choose berries or apples as your snack.

You can even add a little natural nut butter to your apple for a treat. Making small changes, such as these, can get you started on a whole foods plant based diet.

Once you are comfortable swapping out a few snacks, you can start to focus on your three main meals.

Snack Ideas

Many people have the hardest time with switching their snacks over to a whole foods plant based diet. If you think about all of the convenience foods that are available, it can be hard to convince yourself to go that extra step and eat whole foods. Rather than succumbing to preservative and additive laden snacks, take these few simple steps:

- At the beginning of the week chop up plenty of fresh fruits and vegetables and portion them into individual bags. When you want a snack, you can simply grab a bag and go – it's the same as prepackaged food!

- Buy in bulk whenever possible. This allows you to try new whole grains, nuts and seeds and also allows you to make up your own mixes. Don't buy prepackaged trail mix; create your own. Add grains, seeds, nuts, raisins and dates for a truly wonderful and wholesome snack.

- Have plenty of fresh fruit on hand. It's easy to grab an apple, pear or a handful of blueberries. Aside from washing them, there is no other prep work involved.

- Don't get bored. Use hummus, nut butters and salsa to your advantage. Dip your veggies and fruits in them for a little more flavor.

- Keep whole grain tortillas and breads on hand. They can fill you up during those down times and reduce the risk of grabbing that unhealthy candy bar or other sugar laden snack.

Meals

Don't feel overwhelmed at eating a whole foods plant based diet all day long. You might not believe it, but these meals are easier to prepare than the meals you are likely used to eating. Foods that are as close to their source as possible give your body all of its necessary nutrients.

If you keep it simple, meal preparation will actually get easier! Simply choose a whole grain, plenty of vegetables and possibly a starch, such as a sweet potato, and you have a meal.

There's no need for unhealthy additives or condiments. The simpler the choices, the better the meal is for you and the easier it is to prepare.

The key to success is going slow. Don't jump in head first and expect to love the changes. Make a few changes per week to see how your body adjusts.

As you begin to feel the benefits of a whole foods plant based diet you will find yourself wanting to do more.

Think about your food as a way of life or as a way to make your life one that is happy and healthy. Soon enough making the changes will become something that you want to do.

Cooking with Plant Based Whole Foods

Getting Prepared

Before you begin a whole foods plant based diet, determine how you are going to prepare your meals. The more prepared you are, the more likely you will be to actually make this a permanent lifestyle change.

Consider your various cooking methods including:

- Grilling
- Sautéing
- No Cook Meals

Regardless of the method you choose, you can begin to prepare on Sunday for the week ahead. If you plan a week of meals, you can prepare most of the ingredients beforehand.

This only leaves you with final preparation details on a daily basis. Chop up all of your fruits and veggies for the week. Consider the salads you will eat, rice dishes that will include veggies and all of the beans you will need.

Take the time over the weekend to soak your dry beans so that they are ready for cooking right away.

Cooking Grains

Grains are not as time consuming as they sound. All you need to do is boil water, add in your grain of choice, such as quinoa or brown rice and simmer until the liquid has disappeared!

Now you have a good basis for a beautiful plate filled with whole grains topped with delicious vegetables and any spices that you wish to add.

Cooking Beans

Beans require a little more work, which is why it is beneficial to do this preparation once a week to save time. Before you soak your beans, lay them out to locate the bad ones. This also allows you to remove any other particles that might have made their way in there.

The next step involves soaking them. You can do it the overnight way or the quick way:

- **Overnight** – Cover the beans with 3 inches of cold water and cover them. They will need to sit for at least 8 hours, which is why it is considered the overnight method.
- **Quick Method** – If you are in a hurry, you can cover the beans in a pot, with the same amount of water. Bring the water to a boil and leave it for one minute. Then simply remove the beans from the heat, letting them sit covered for one hour.

After draining your soaked beans, you will cover them with 2 inches of water and add any spices or an onion that you want to add for flavor.

Bring the water to a boil and let them simmer, covered for the next 1 to 1 ½ hours.

No Cook Meals

It is easy to get away with meals that do not require any cooking when you follow a whole foods plant based diet. Think about the many salads you can make.

Even if you ate them several times per week, simply switching up the veggies that you put on top of your salad will make it seem like a completely different meal.

You could even get creative and add nuts, seeds or even a small amount of whole grain pasta to give your salads a little texture.

Fast Meals

Every family is busy and runs into those days that no one has time to sit at the table and eat a meal. Don't resort to convenience foods during these times. Be prepared with foods already made in the freezer, such as:

- Bean burritos made with whole grain tortillas
- Potatoes with a few spices can make a quick meal
- Sweet potatoes provide even more nutrition
- Find your favorite recipe for veggie burgers and make them in bulk to have on hand in the freezer
- A handful of fruits and nuts are always a good way to fill up on healthy food

- Soup can also be made in bulk and stocked full with veggies. Freeze the leftovers for a quick meal.

Eating a whole foods plant based diet requires a little dedication and the desire to want to live a long, happy life.

Whether you adopt one of the techniques talked about in the book or all of them, any change is good for your health.

Take it slow as you figure out what you and your family like and then you can have a successful transition to a whole foods plant based diet!

Made in the USA
Lexington, KY
13 March 2014